Pocket Guide to
Back Pain

GW00694279

Pocket Guide to

Back Pain

Anthony G. Reed FIPA MCam

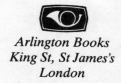

Arlington Books
King St, St James's
London

POCKET GUIDE TO BACK PAIN
Second Edition first published 1989 by
Arlington Books (Publishers) Ltd
15–17 King St, St James's
London SW1

First edition published 1982

© Anthony G. Reed 1982, 1989

British Library Cataloguing-in-Publication Data

Reed, Anthony G.
    Pocket guide to back pain. – 2nd ed.
    1. Man. Back. Backache
    I. Title
    616.7'3

    ISBN 0–85140–756–0

Typeset by TJB Photosetting, Grantham
Printed and bound in Great Britain by
Richard Clay Ltd, Bungay

About the Author

ANTHONY G. REED FIPA MCam qualified as a writer and for many years operated his own group of publicity companies on technical subjects. He then turned to publishing and launched a magazine on the River Thames and two other magazines, one for an Area Health Authority. For several years he also assisted the National Back Pain Association as their Information Officer and Training Officer, editing their magazine. He has written many published articles and training manuals regarding all aspects of back pain and its avoidance.

Contents

Introduction

The human back can be seen as a very complicated piece of engineering permitting flexible movement of the body and limbs in all directions, whilst carrying all the essential communications between the brain and the various parts of the body. The spine itself, whilst supporting the body against the downward pressure of gravity and carrying all the nerves that serve to communicate feeling and movement, is an amazing series of mechanical facets held together by elastic muscles, ligaments and tendons.

It is not surprising, therefore, that within this organisation there are many sources for failure causing pain, each with a variety of possible causes. For simplicity all these failures and resulting sensations are brought together under one heading – Back Pain, which is now an accepted definition both nationally and by the World Health Organisation.

Covering as it does such a wide variety of causes and effects, back pain now has an increasing number of specialists investigating and learning about this interesting part of the body, which until quite recently had been given little attention because of the difficulties involved.

Many books and papers have been written on the subject, but invariably of a learned nature, and far beyond the comprehension of the layman. It is for this reason that this book has been written. The majority of us will suffer back pain in some form during our lives and because if we know more about how to use our backs correctly we could avoid much of this back pain, it is important that we should understand the problem.

So, using layman's language, with a simplification that the medical profession may find mundane, it is hoped that at last a greater understanding of the back will lead to less back pain. The more we understand of a problem the more we can take preventive action.

Chapter 1
Back Pain, A Major Problem

Until fairly recently, to suffer from back pain was considered by others to be a source of amusement, and was frequently regarded with suspicion by employers as an excuse for malingering.

In the past few years however, as more has become known about the back, how it works and the problems that can arise, a more serious attitude has been taken on what many specialists have come to realise is one of the greatest scourges of mankind today.

Statistics are now supplied by the Department of Health and Social Security, linked to the World Health Organisation's international classification of diseases. Limited to certain categories of back pain and classifications of people, and therefore representing only a small part of the overall suffering, these statistics have nevertheless surprised many people and continue to show an increase. It is estimated that four out of five people in the UK will suffer back pain to some degree during their lives. A similar proportion is also given for America and most civilised nations.

Due to the attention brought to the problem of spinal ailments by the National Back Pain Association supported by many of the medical and other professions, Government departments are beginning to realise that it is a serious, and very costly problem for the nation. In any year the number of cases of certified illness due to back pain will be around 20 million a year, and industry loses the services of more than 80,000 people every day. In lost production, and cost to the Health Service, this represents a loss of over £1,000 million every year. It is no wonder that these ailments are now receiving more attention by Government and industry, yet for every £100 spent on medical research in this country, only 7p is allocated to back pain research.

In the mining industry back pain is now accepted as being the greatest cause for absenteeism, even greater than silicosis. It is probably in this field that the most early research was carried out to reduce the high incidence of back pain. By the use of the ultrasonic scanner it was found that a considerable variation occurred in the dimension of different people's spinal cord (the tunnel in the centre of the spine through which the nerves pass), and by measuring this it became possible to improve the selection of miners for work on the face of the mine less prone to spinal problems. In the nursing profession the manual movement of patients causes over 40,000 trained nurses to be absent from their essential service every year due to back problems. Similarly here with nurses, research instigated by the NBPA (National Back Pain Association) into lifting techniques, with the co-operation of Surrey University and the Royal College of Nursing, enabled a Manual on the Handling of Patients to be produced which is now used as the basis for all nurse training and is making this movement of patients a less hazardous operation.

In 1979 a report to the Secretary of State for Social Services by a working party on back pain set up under Professor A.L. Cochrane, stated: There is a profound and widespread dissatisfaction with what is at present available to help people who suffer from back pain. However, the evidence on most approaches to treatment is unsatisfactory and often conflicting, largely due to the fact that most forms of therapy have not been evaluated in an acceptable and scientific manner.

It is generally accepted that one of the major problems associated with back pain is the variety of causes, some interrelated and others not, and that insufficient knowledge has been collected as a result of research to enable medical practitioners to always make an accurrate diagnosis of the cause for particular suffering.

As more is learnt about spinal ailments however, one factor has become apparent; much of the loss to the nation, and the suffering, could be avoided if people were better educated about using their bodies, and especially their spines.

Chapter 2
Probable Causes
of Back Pain

In the past it was suggested that we suffer because the spine was not originally created to accept man in an upright position, and that the spine has not developed sufficiently since the apeman travelled on all fours or swung from branch to branch in the trees.

Scientists have now disproven this theory by making comparisons with the spinal patterns of other animals. The force of gravity is a problem for all animals, but this gravitational force on upright or vertical animals is far less than on one that is always horizontal, as can be seen with the dipping spine of ageing horses and donkeys.

Man's spine has evolved and it is a marvel of biological engineering, designed for maximum movement where most necessary (neck and trunk), with thicker bones to give greater strength at the base (lumber region above the buttocks) ending at the *coccyx* (where the tail used to be).

The most likely reason for the present high level of back suffering is that we misuse our spines today due to the types of lives which we lead. In the wildness of Africa and South America, where man still accepts a very basic life style with plenty of exercise and movement, spinal ailments – other than through accidental damage – are almost unknown. Let us look at the soft, easy life enjoyed by civilized man (which includes women in all respects). We see little exercise, little muscular movement or development and a general sagging appearance of our bodies most of the time. We sit for long periods in ill-designed chairs, we drive around in cars or sit in public vehicles, and also we subject parts of our spine to sudden stresses when turning, reaching and lifting. It is not surprising that we suffer when we misuse our spines so badly.

The major problem with back pain is that it can be caused by a very large number of different ailments, some mechanical and others chemical. Fortunately, few result in serious or permanent disability, and as more becomes known about this most intricate part of our body, new methods for diagnosis and treatment are being found. Back pain is not emotive, as are cancer or heart disease – except to the sufferer himself – and nobody is likely to die from it, although many cases of suicide have been identified as being caused by the continuous debilitating pain that some forms of backache can cause.

Knowing today that apart from accidental damage, most of the spinal ailments can be avoided by using our bodies correctly, we should be persuaded to do something about it and so cope with the problem.

The spine is a most complex piece of engineering. We should always remember this and think about it before subjecting the spine to extra stresses. We should think about standing up straight, sitting up straight, walking upright, making smooth movements without sudden jerks, not to carry heavy loads and to keep our spine at all times in the shape it was meant to be (see *Figure 1* for the slight 'S' shape of the spine). If we do take care we stand a better chance of living a normal active life without incurring excruciating pain.

It must also be understood that as we become older our body degenerates. This degeneration, from the age of thirty-five to forty years onwards, is a natural result of the ageing process, but the extent to which our spine will degenerate, and the trouble and pain that we may suffer as a result, will depend on how we have used or abused it when we were younger, in our more active years.

Chapter 3
The Back, Its Construction and Purpose

Let us take a careful look at this natural architectural masterpiece, the spine (Fig. 1.).

It is made up of 33 separate bones (*vertebrae*) sculptured to fit each other, of which 24 are separated by discs acting like combined shock-absorbers and pivots, permitting movement in different directions. They are all held together by an intricate pattern of muscles, tendons and ligaments, so forming the scaffold upon which the rest of the body performs (See Fig. 3.).

The spine withstands forces of hundreds of pounds, yet is so flexible that it can be turned through 90° in any direction or bent over to form two-thirds of a circle. Right through the centre of this column (the spinal cord) are threaded the nerves which carry the messages to and from the brain to operate every part of the body.

Although flexible in all directions, all the parts are held in delicate balance so that damage to one part can disrupt the whole. Pressure on the nerves at one part of the spine can cause pain remote from the seat

Figure 1

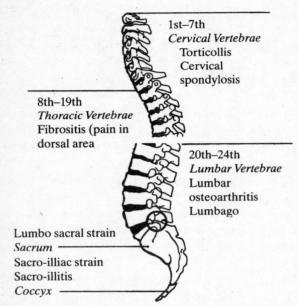

1st–7th
Cervical Vertebrae
  Torticollis
  Cervical
  spondylosis

8th–19th
Thoracic Vertebrae
Fibrositis (pain in
dorsal area

20th–24th
Lumbar Vertebrae
Lumbar
osteoarthritis
Lumbago

Lumbo sacral strain
Sacrum
Sacro-illiac strain
Sacro-illitis
Coccyx

The upper and lower parts of the spine, showing the vertebrae separated by the discs (solid black) and some of the ailments resulting from failures.

of the trouble, perhaps in the hands and arms from damage at the neck, or feet and legs from damage in the lumbar region (above the buttocks).

The All-Important Discs

The visco-elastic discs which separate the bones and permit their flexibility of movement, are a most important part of the spine and are often the cause of many of our problems. These discs (*inter-vertebrae discs*) have a tough outer body with a soft jelly centre. The tension of this jelly centre is dependent upon a balance of fluid pressure (just like hydraulic shock-absorbers). This fluid is absorbed from the surrounding tissues during the night whilst we are asleep, and squeezed out during the day when the discs are constantly withstanding the force of gravity as the bones (*vertebrae*) press down on them. The greater this pres-

Figure 2

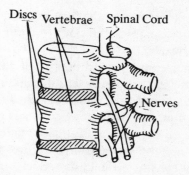

Discs Vertebrae Spinal Cord

Nerves

The vertebrae, *separated by discs, with the spinal cord running through the column and nerves branching out to enter arms, legs, etc., through apertures in the column.*

sure, such as additional loads being put onto the spine by lifting heavy weights, the greater the loss of fluid. All of us are a fraction taller in the morning than we are at the end of day, due to the amount of fluid held in the discs. When gravity is eliminated, as with the weightlessness experienced by astronauts, the hydrostatic pressure is reduced, and the astronauts return to earth several centimetres taller than when they left, temporarily.

The damaged disc is a common cause of backache, as a result of undue stress being put upon it, often caused by lifting excessive loads or lifting when the spine is bent or turned. There is no such thing as a 'slipped' disc. What often happens is that the shock-absorbing discs give way, allowing the jelly part (the *nucleus*) to bulge out. If this bulge presses against one of the spinal nerves the result is pain, and often excruciating pain at the point of pressure or in the limbs served by that nerve.

Another common and important cause of pain is from damage to the muscle fibres and ligaments that hold the spine in position. When the body moves the muscles contract. If the movement is rapid or jerky, especially if the muscle is already under tension, the muscles may be strained or the fibres tear, and pain results at the site of the failure. Such damage will usually get better fairly quickly if rested and not subjected to additional stress.

The bones of the back are held together by tough

Figure 3

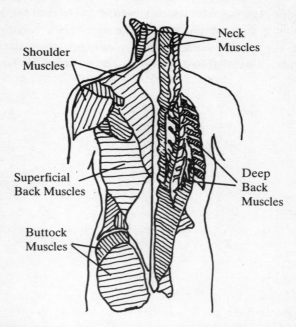

Shoulder
Muscles

Neck
Muscles

Superficial
Back Muscles

Deep
Back
Muscles

Buttock
Muscles

The main muscles affecting the spine, which play an important part in the mechanism of the back.

ligaments and tendons. These too can be torn if subjected to too much or too sudden a movement. Here again they may repair themselves quite quickly if given the chance, although ligaments have a poor blood supply so the recovery may be delayed.

It is also worth mentioning pain caused by muscle spasms, as these can cause a vicious circle. Relatively minor damage can cause a muscle spasm and set up a pain 'circuit' which can be difficult to break, and many patients who have suffered one of these minor attacks of back pain often develop disc problems later.

Chapter 4
Pain is Subjective

Pain is personal. It cannot be measured. It is a subjective psychological experience in which only the sufferer can take part. Only the sufferer knows the extent of the pain, although methods have now been found to record it.

One of the sad facts about backache is that the pain is often severe, and can be continuous. Pain caused by an impingement upon a nerve is different to muscular pain, but it is difficult to explain such differences when the nature of all pain is personal. It is insufficient to say that nerve pain is sharp and muscle pain dull, as such terms mean different things to different people. Hence differences in type of pain can seldom be used to assist in diagnosing the cause.

As has been seen, the spine carries right down its centre the spinal cord, which is an extension of the brain, and from it nerve roots extend to all parts of the body. So that in addition to inflammation or damage to the spine itself, its muscles, ligaments and tendons, the nerves can become compressed by the discs or the bones themselves. The whole area is highly sensitive, with several interrelated activities, and identifying the source of any trouble is extremely difficult. The use of modern equipment such as X-rays, myelograms (the injection of dyes into the spinal column), CAT scanners (expensive computerised X-ray scanners) or diasonographs (ultrasonic measuring scanners) enables more to be seen of the bonal structure of the spine, but no method of seeing the discs, muscles or ligaments has yet been found. Fortunately, the bones of the spine are near the skin surface in the back which enables those disciplines who practise manipulation (osteopaths, chiropactors, with some physiotherapists and doctors) by sensitive finger investigation of the bone structure, its flexibility and movement, to identify some of the failures which may be causing the pain. Today, too, referred pain (pain at different site to the failure) is more widely understood, so that pain in arms and hands, legs and feet, can be identified as being caused by pressure on the nerve at specifice vertebrae and joints of the spine, and thus the necessary corrective treatment attempted.

The gaps in the *vertebrae* through which the nerves pass are small. They become smaller when the spine is bent or turned, hence the nerves are more likely to suffer, and give pain, when stress is added to a bent or turned back. A slight squeezing of the nerve results in a 'pins and needles' sensation in hands, arms, feet or legs, which may develop into severe pain if that pressure increases.

The support of the muscles plays a large part in this action. If the muscles are slack (due to lack of exercise or degeneration with age) they will give less support. Similarly, general stress and worry can cause the shoulder muscles to contract (giving a hunched appearance), and if at the same time additional stress caused by lifting or turning quickly is imposed, damage is more likely to occur. Often with pain, the muscles themselves, in a protective manner, will contract automatically at the site of the failure (go into a spasm) with the result that the back will seize up, and no movement whatever is possible until the muscles relax again. This often happens with *lumbago*, and there is nothing so frightening as to bend down to pick something up and — pain, excruciating pain, is felt in the back and all movement is frozen, often in the bent position. One is completely paralysed (with all its connotations). What has happened is that the muscle, as an automatic preventive measure, has gone into a spasm. This will probably ease with time and rest, and yet there will seem to be no reason for this severe attack.

It has been found that backache is often a cumulative process. Stresses will be imposed on the spine a number of times without any suffering, often over a long period of time. Then later, a slight movement will be 'the last straw' and severe pain will develop, probably with muscle spasm.

From all these somewhat simplified explanations of the working of the spine, and the problems that can occur, it can be appreciated that diagnosis becomes a very difficult task for many medical practitioners, but is essential before successful treatment can be recommended.

Chapter 5
Some Common Back Pain Complaints

Strained or Torn Ligaments and Muscles
When a spinal joint is sprained badly, the ligaments which support the joint structure and control the range of movements, can be stretched or torn. The result is immediate pain at the site of the damage which often increases in the days following. If rest is taken, then the ligament or tendon damage will repair itself. If however, the activity which caused the damage is continued then a serious weakening may occur, resulting in permanent damage and more chronic pain.

Such damage can be caused by a simple act of stretching too far or too quickly, turning or bending quickly or jerkily, lifting heavy weights incorrectly or remaining in a bent position or sitting without support to the back for long periods – or a combination of any or all of these actions. Even a sudden cough or sneeze when the body is badly sited may cause minor damage. Subjecting the spine to continuous strain by obesity or poor posture can also eventually strain a ligament.

Muscle damage has similar causes, and effects, being the tearing of the muscle fibres. Incorrect lifting especially can cause immediate tearing of muscle fibres with pain resulting at the site of the damage. Fortunately rest and keeping reasonably warm will permit the fibres to repair themselves.

These sprains and tears are probably the most common sources of backache, hence rest and the use of pain-killing drugs are usually the first treatments recommended by the medical practitioner, and in most cases the damage will be cured naturally.

Adhesions

Nature has a way of repairing many inflammations automatically, by causing a sticky fluid to be formed at the site of any inflammation. Unfortunately in many cases this fluid can stick one adjacent surface to another, and fibrous tissues will form. With a sprained ankle and the formation of such tissues, exercise or walking will restore mobility. When such adhesions, or lesions as they are sometimes called, form on the spine, they may cause two surfaces in this complicated area to adhere, and the tendency is not to move at all as movement causes pain. With such lesions, exercise, or in some cases, manipulation, is usually recommended which will free the adhered joints. Lesions, therefore, require completely different treatment from sprained ligaments and muscles hence osteopaths, chiropractors and many physiotherapists and doctors now practise manipulation.

Disc Displacement or Protrusion

As has been seen, putting too much stress on the *intervertebral discs* (between the *vertebrae*) can cause them to become displaced; the *nucleus* (the jelly centre) being squeezed out and protruding against the spinal cord or the nerve root, which is often incorrectly referred to as 'a slipped disc'. Figure 4 illustrates a prolapsed disc, with the nucleus being pressed out against the nerve, often resulting in referred pain at some other site, at the leg, arm, etc., as well as the site of the damage.

This can be brought about by degeneration, when the disc becomes shallower, or by stress such as lifting heavy weights incorrectly, or subjecting the spine to a bad jolt, and can produce considerable pain. It occurs most commonly in the lumbar region (just above the buttocks), and the prolapse, as the protrusion is called, can occur long after the stress has been imposed or as a result of cumulative stress. A sudden movement like bending down to pick up a pin, or by coughing and sneezing, would then result in sudden pain. It may be so severe that the muscle also goes into spasm and the body cannot be straightened. Absolute bed rest is required, traction (stretching of the spine), manipulation or the wearing of special jackets and corsets may be necessary over a long period, before the disc returns to a healthier state. It is doubtful if the

Figure 4

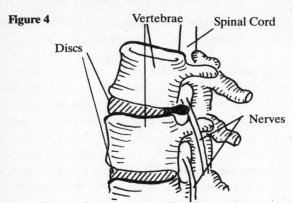

The prolapsed disc. Compare this illustration of the vertebrae and discs with Fig. 2. Here pressure has been placed downwards on the disc whilst bending and turning – the outer skin of the disc has burst open and the nucleus has bulged out pressing on to the nearby nerve, causing severe pain here and possibly also in the legs or arms.

disc ever returns to normality although a 'second rate' repair may occur.

Degenerative Changes

It has already been stated that the body degenerates with age, and the spine can degenerate in different ways depending upon the stresses to which it has been subjected in earlier days.

It should be stated immediately that normal degeneration of the spine can occur from forty years of age up to seventy, without any suffering whatsoever. The natural flattening or compression of the discs often causes the spine to shrink, especially if the muscles have been allowed to become slack through lack of use, and the natural height of that person reduces in later life. The spine also becomes stiffer with old age and therefore more care is needed to avoid heavy lifting, quick movements connected with turning or bending or long periods spent in the same position. There is a greater need for exercise to keep the spine flexible and the muscles in good condition.

Degenerative changes occur a great deal earlier for those engaged in heavy manual work, or those whose spine has suffered many shocks due to sport or similar activity.

Spondylosis is the term for the deterioration caused by such degeneration (not to be confused with *spondylitis*, which is the inflammation of the joints of the spine). *Cervical spondylosis*, affecting the neck, is a fairly common malaise causing stiffness, or protrusions and lesions being formed on the *cervical vertebrae*. The nerves passing from the spinal cord through the small channels in the bone can become compressed or diverted by these small formations of new bone. This "wear and tear" of the neck structure can result in headaches, spreading from the neck over the top of the head, or pain in the neck, arms and hands. These can be mere sensations such as 'pins and needles' or acute pain. After rest, traction or manipulation, they often disappear within a few weeks but may reappear sometime later.

Similarly, *lumbar spondylosis* may occur at the

lower end of the spine, causing pain in the lumbar region and in the legs. When this happens difficulty can be experienced throughout the day and especially at night when sleeping, as the neck and body becomes twisted into odd postures so that pain results either then or the following morning.

Strangely enough, it appears that symptoms from *spondylosis* occur more often in the thirty to fifty age group than in the elderly. Providing steps are taken to relieve acute pain by the use of drugs, and when necessary, physiotherapy and regular exercise as directed by the medical team, *spondylosis* can be lived with in a normal manner. However, once *spondylosis* has developed it does not disappear, although the symptoms may.

Spondylosis, which is seldom serious, is often confused with *osteoarthritis*, as both can be caused by normal degeneration. Whilst *spondylosis* affects the *vertebrae* and discs, *osteoarthritis* affects only the smaller joints and therefore is found at the top of the neck (*cervical* joints) and the lower part of the spine (lowest two *lumbar* joints). The two conditions are however, interrelated. *Spondylosis* appears at an earlier stage of degeneration of the spine than *osteoarthritis*, and both appear to be the result of disc degeneration.

Osteoarthritis may cause continuous pain, varying in severity from time to time, and more commonly affects those over sixty, with the condition worsening with age. It does also, of course, affect other joints such as the hips and knees.

Deformation

The most common causes of backache have now been dealt with, and those that remain are far more rare.

Spinal curvatures, as a result of disease or at birth, sometimes lead to pain, but those major abnormal curvatures which have been caused by injury invariably lead to painful experience if they are not corrected.

Scoliosis is the sideways bending of the spine. Few people have perfectly straight spines (or more correctly, a perfect 'S' shape,) and a slight sideways bend is unlikely to cause any discomfort. A slight postural *scoliosis* is very different in all respects from a major deformity which will invariably require surgery to straighten the spine.

Lordosis, the hollow back resulting from obesity or slack abdominal muscles, is often suffered by women in pregnancy as a result of trying to balance the extra weight of the child in the womb. Again it is not likely to cause much permanent backache unless it leads to early degenerative changes. In later life as the discs become narrower, there is a risk of the nerves being squeezed and pain may develop. The oposite form to *lordosis* is *kyphosis*, or round back (hunchback), which is often caused by disease, such as *tuberculosis* of the spine or *osteochondrosis*, the latter often being hereditary. It may also be caused by poor working posture when leaning over a work area for very long periods, and especially tall people are more prone. In later years this also can lead to greater immobility and resulting back pain.

Spondylolisthesis means the slipping forward of the upper spine onto the *vertebrae* below, usually as the result of an injury or bad jarring, as with a fall or jump. It can also be hereditary. Showing clearly on X-rays (unlike many other forms of back trouble) it can cause pain due to pressure on nerve roots. If in the *sacrum* (centre of the buttocks), a frequent site for such a fracture, it can result in some disablement or discomfort.

Psychosomatic Back Pain

Finally, back trouble can be psychosomatic. In industry back pain has often been accused of being an easy method of malingering. Specialists report however, that malingering with back pain is very rare as there is always a basis of pain to some degree.

As has been shown, pain is subjective, and one person's pain cannot be experienced or easily imagined by another.

Back troubles can become worse as a result of other forms of stress, whether emotional or physical. Pain is also harder to bear if the sufferer worries, about a job, the family or finance. Pain itself is depressing, and continuous pain as experienced with some forms of back trouble can cause severe depression.

It has often been noted that a back pain sufferer finds that the pain becomes worse when he can least afford the time to obtain treatment, because of heavy business demands or family pressures.

Psychosomatic back trouble is a fact, and as with headaches, the source of the trouble should be sought rather than waiting for repeated sessions of pain whenever stress of some kind is experienced. The answer to this form of back trouble is seldom found in pain-killing drugs.

We have noted that when a person is suffering stress, worry or even anger, he will often stand with hunched shoulders indicating a tightening of the muscles. It is when muscles are taut that damage can most easily occur. Such action can even cause contraction of the *cervical* spine at the neck, which in the event of lesions or disc damage, will cause pain as a result of pressure on the nerve roots.

Chapter 6
Avoiding Back Pain

Having identified some of the many causes of back pain, is it possible to avoid all this pain, even in today's indolent society?

Since the most common causes can be identified, and these represent perhaps 90% of backache problems, it would appear that if we learnt to live with some consideration of our back, we would have a very good chance of avoiding much pain, and the loss of work which often results. With a little care we could also avoid many of the accidents which damage the spine.

With backache, **prevention is certainly far better than possible cure**, and can result from more knowledge about our body, especially our spine, and how not to misuse it.

So let us look at the steps that can be taken. They are, in the main, very simple, and if we can remember them, and **think back** before we act, we can beat this modern malady.

Sitting, Standing and Walking Correctly.
The spine is never still. It moves with every breath we take. Breathe in deeply and the *thoracic* section of the spine (behind the ribs and lungs) straightens. Breathe out and it flexes forward.

Remember that gravity imposes a constant force on us all the time, and on our spine. This gravitational force on the spine is at its least when we lie down. So quite logically, if we could lie down more we would put less stress on our spine. This is worth remembering when we have a chance to relax. We would do so better in the supine position, preferably lying on the floor or a firm base – or even better in the 'Psoas' position, with the feet and legs raised on a stool. Some schools of thought in America even go so far as to suggest that we should stand on our heads against the wall to reverse the force of gravity, although many others think that this could be rather hazardous, especially for back pain sufferers.

Since, however, we do have to stand, sit and move about, let us do it as sensibly as possible, conscious that it is our spine that permits our movements, and it must therefore be considered all the time. If we develop correct postural habits we will protect our spine naturally.

Posture and Deportment
The Victorians had strong views about posture and deportment. Young ladies were made to balance a

book on their heads as they walked ensuring an upright position with a straight spine, so providing minimal stress and area for gravitational force. Stomach and chin held in combined with perfect balance. Slouching was strictly forbidden. This is the ideal attitude and one we should all strive for.

We then come to a very important point to watch – our weight. We cannot create a good posture if we are flabby and fat, if our stomach sticks out so that we are bent forward to cope with it making our spine permanently curved. Obesity is considered by many to be a major factor in the cause of backache. With this obesity we also have natural degeneration with age causing a stiffening of the spine with shrinking discs. We therefore invite trouble if extra weight, especially in the stomach, is adding stress to the gravitational force. Thus, if for no other reason than avoiding back-ache, we should keep fit, keep muscles flexible by exercise and keep our weight down.

Bad Habits at an Early Age

As children we are taught many things, but seldom are we taught how to stand and walk, It is taken for granted that this is a natural process, but bad habits can develop early. More thought should be given at school in teaching children good posture, good deportment and how to sit up straight.

Even before he walks a baby crawls on all fours or pulls himself along, seated on the floor. Later he moves himself along with one leg bent underneath, propelling himself with the other leg in a series of bumps. These bumps are on the buttocks, jolting the spine. Such movements should be discouraged, and at least ensure that the baby wears a thick nappy to cushion these shocks. Such care becomes more important with his first steps before falling back into the sitting position, when even greater shock can be given to the developing spine. The use of a baby 'walking machine' can avoid much of this.

As the child grows up and habits form, correct posture should be taught both in the home and at school. Walk tall and sit up straight. Again we must quote our Victorian forebears who also emphasised a correct sitting position – initially training children to sit with arms folded behind the back for short periods, so forming a hollow back with a straight spine. Children may not react well to such training but it can make such a difference later, so constant reminders may be necessary. A good mnemonic is 'S U S', "Sit up Straight" or "Stand up Straight", to be stated whenever a child (or grown-up, for that matter) is seen standing or walking with shoulders hunched, or slouching in a chair.

At school, unfortunately, many desks today have not been properly designed to give support to the lumbar region of the back, which should be combined with a sloping writing area to encourage upright sitting, as they were in the past. The modern trend is for the use of tables and chairs planned to suit all ages and sizes, which they cannot do. Instead they encourage slouching forward to write with bent backs, so storing up trouble for the children in later years. All we can do is to keep pressing for better design, with the correct size of desk and chair to cope with the growing child.

Children Learn by Example

We should set a good example for our children to follow in the home. They should see us with good posture and deportment, never hunched up or slouching about.

We should have furniture designed to cope with our bodies correctly, and with items placed conveniently around the house so that we avoid stretching, bending and lifting.

Chairs should have straight backs to encourage sitting up straight, with the seat at a height that keeps the knees above the seat and feet just on the ground. Easy chairs should have straight backs with padding to support the lumbar region. Many modern, so called 'comfortable' easy chairs make it virtually impossible to sit properly, especially when the seat is very soft or deep. 'Bucket' type chairs should always be avoided.

As we sit for many hours these days watching television, it is important that we do not slouch in the chair or settee. It may seem that we are relaxed, but if the spine is in a twisted state for a long period, and we then get up quickly, we are likely to suffer some damage to the back. Even a sneeze or cough, when we are hunched up or twisted, can produce backache – not necessarily at the time, but at some period afterwards.

Coughing at any time can cause stress on the chest muscles, and on the spine, hence smoking, which often causes coughing, is not conducive to a good spinal condition.

Always avoid quick jerky movements. Try to rise from the chair, or the bed, in a smooth flowing movement, and then walk with a smooth progression.

Stand erect, but avoid standing still for long periods. If it is necessary, change the weight from one foot to the other, from time to time. Sway backwards and sideways occasionally to maintain flexibility.

Ergonomics in the Home

Ergonomics, the science of planning the environment for the activities involved to the best effect, is used in the office and factory. It can be just as important in the home to avoid backache.

Let us therefore look at the furniture and fitments throughout the house. Could everyday activities be carried out with less stretching, less bending and less stress? Are all the work surfaces at the best height so that we can stand, or sit upright, without bending over? The correct position for a work surface is a few inches below the elbow. For a tall person it may be advisable to place blocks of wood under the sink unit to raise it, so that the many hours spent at the sink do not create a curved back.

It may cost more to have a split-level oven, but it does avoid stooping down to lift out heavy dishes – If this has to be done from a low oven, bend the knees and lower to a squatting position, lifting out the meat dish by straightening the legs and keeping the back straight. Never turn at the same time as lifting a heavy object.

All the items in the kitchen in regular use should be kept in cupboards or on shelves at a height which will avoid bending or stretching. If high cupboards have to be used, stand on a small pair of household steps (never on a chair which can topple over), and do not try and reach up from the floor without squatting first.

With household cleaning try to vacuum under furniture without bending, keeping the handle of the machine close to the body. Wash floors by kneeling on a mat, not bending over. Try not to bend over when making a bed – go round to the other side and kneel down to keep the back straight. Do not try turning a mattress by yourself. It is a very difficult load to handle; always get help.

Plan your actions in the home so as not to put stress on your spine. Once you have planned the work well, it will not take long for you to develop good habits.

Mothers at Risk
Mothers of babies and young children are particularly

susceptible to backache, caused by bad movements. When stomach and back muscles have not fully re-covered from pregnancy and childbirth, she finds that she has to lift baby, weighing several pounds, in and out of a low cot, bath and pram many times a day. There will be no strain on the spine if the lifting is done by bending the knees and not the back. Keep as close to the cot as possible and lift or replace the baby by bending arms and knees, keeping the back straight. When carrying the baby, the child should be held close to the body, not out at arms length when the force on the spine is many times the child's weight. As the child becomes larger and heavier take particular care when lifting him off the floor. It is so easy, when in a hurry, to bend down and pick up the child without thinking, and then perhaps some time later, backache develops. The strain should always be taken by the legs and not the back.

The worst thing to do is to bend over, lift a heavy weight and then turn or twist the body. Turning or twisting the spine when it is under stress squeezes the discs and greatly increases the risk of disc lesion or torn ligaments, as so many people will bear witness having suffered intense pain as a result of a simple act of lifting incorrectly. Even carrying a heavy shopping bag can be a risk. Whenever possible, the load should be broken down into two shopping bags of equal weight to balance either side of the body. Take care too when unloading a supermarket trolley at the cash desk. It is difficult to do without bending over.

Another common act which can cause heavy stress is lifting packages, or baby, out of the back of a car from the front seat. In the confined space the lifting has to be done at arms length and the body turned at the same time, both actions being dangerous for the spine. Similarly, lifting packages from the car boot is fraught with danger if it is a deep boot. Far better with a 'hatch back' when the load can be slid to the rear and then lifted with legs slightly bent.

The heavier the weight lifted, the greater the stress on the spine. See if the weight can be broken down into a number of smaller loads – if not, can someone give assistance?

Chapter 7
Lifting is a Major Cause of Back Pain

We have dealt with some of the lifting problems in the home. Lifting heavy objects is one of the greatest causes of backache, for as we saw when we considered the mechanics of the spine, extra pressure is put upon the discs and if squeezed too much, especially when bent or turned, they will bulge and possibly fracture or create displacements resulting in considerable pain, at the site of the damage or in the legs and arms.

What then is a safe weight to lift?

No load is 'safe'. Bulky and unstable loads are far more dangerous than compact and stable ones with a handle or some protrusion which can be grasped. However, people should be discouraged from attempting to lift loads which exceed half their own body weight, possibly one third for women. If it feels heavy when you test it, do not attempt to lift it – get help.

Frequently lifting is an occupational hazard, and considerable steps are taken by some companies to train their staff in the correct methods to be used in order to avoid back trouble. The same hazards are there in the home, garden and office. If lifting heavy objects has to be carried out, and it is done correctly, the risk of damage is considerably reduced. In many cases it is a question of 'teaching old dogs new tricks' because we all feel that we know how to lift objects, but those new tricks will avoid the risk of much pain.

In the factory, it has become so important for workers to be trained correctly on lifting that legislation has now been enacted to ensure that management arranges for this training, and that workers do carry out what they are taught. In fact, the EEC has made manual handling a matter for directives to be issued throughout Europe. The principles involved in safe manual handling in the factory are equally important in the office, laboratory and other places of work. Agricultural workers are particularly at risk with the manual handling of heavy sacks and other difficult loads. Many training aids are used by management, including a Material Handling Manual, with a series of posters, supplied by the NBPA.

Some Basic Lifting Rules
The first rule is to plan the lift carefully. Look at it to see if it can be simplified. Can the load be broken down into a number of lighter loads? Can the lift be taken in stages, from the floor to a bench, and then from the bench to the final site? Is there any mechanical help available, such as a rope and pulley, or can it

be slid up a plank? Is assistance available?

When the method has been carefully considered, here are some basic rules:

Figure 5

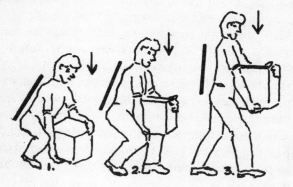

1 Stand over the load with feet apart, the load equidistant between the feet.
2 Bend the hips and knees to get down to the level of the load. Do NOT get down onto one knee.
3 Keep the back in a straight line from head to tail.
4 Grip the load firmly with both hands, preferably with one hand below the object.
5 Keep arms close to the body, with the load also as close to the body as is possible.
6 Look over the load to ensure that there are no potential hazards ahead, steps, boxes, etc.
7 Using thigh and leg muscles, lift the load smoothly.

8 It may be possible to use motion to ease the lift, by creating a slight swinging action backwards and lifting as the load comes forward, in one fluid movement. (This is the basis of kinetic handling, using the weight of the load to help its movement, and it is very useful with some types of load.)

9 Having lifted the load to an upright position, stand straight with the load close to the body. Walk forward and do not twist the body.

10 If the load feels too heavy, put it down onto a table or back on the floor if there is no convenient alternative, and take a rest.

11 When lowering the load, reverse the action by bending hips and knees until you have lowered the load to the ground, still maintaining a straight back.

NOTE: If after testing, you do lift the load but then find it too heavy, put it down onto the ground again and seek help – it is better than getting backache.

There may seem to be a large number of rules to remember, but they are very simple and once a correct lift has been used several times, the movements will come more easily. Beware of emergencies, when the tendency is to return to bad habits – and possible backache. The important thing to remember is to keep the back straight. When the back is bent, the extra pressure put onto the discs is equal to the weight of the load plus two thirds of the body weight, multiplied by six. Too much for anyone's discs.

Several difficult types of load need special handling – rolls of carpet, long planks, drums, etc. For advice on these special loads and how to handle them the National Back Pain Association have produced special posters, a lifting guide and a training manual (see page 64).

Figure 6

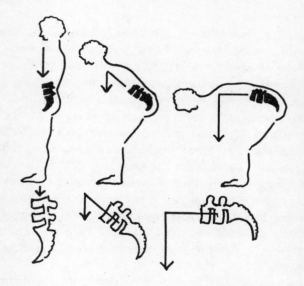

The diagrams show the increasing pressure exerted on to the vertebrae and discs, with their surrounding muscles and tendons, when bending. The fulcrum effect multiplies the pressure with movement from the vertical, to which should be added any weights lifted or carried.

Chapter 8
Occupational Hazards

We have mentioned the special hazards in many industrial occupations, but as well as manual workers the back can also be at risk in the office and with more sedentary occupations. Reaching and stretching for files and books after long periods sitting at a desk, crouched over ledgers, bad posture and badly designed furniture can all lead to back problems. Whilst on the whole typist's chairs are well designed to give some support for the lumbar region of the back during the many hours she sits there, she also has to constantly bend and twist her neck to read the copy being typed, all creating stress. Raised and angled reading stands could do much to help her, and all those who need to read or refer to books and documents.

Occupational hazards also occur in our normal pursuits in the home, garden and many leisure activities.

Just as miners, construction workers, warehousemen and nurses have to be trained to do their work without incurring back troubles, so do those of us who lift shopping, children and baggage, dig and lift heavy soil, carry sacks, shovel coal or saw logs – we all put our backs at risk.

When we are young our muscles are strong, our spines are flexible and well supported. We can play sports, football, rugby and row with accidents being the only cause for backache – at the time. These activities could however, be the source for back problems later in life. But as we become less flexible in later years, occupational hazards in and around the home have to be considered more carefully.

Do-it-yourself enthusiasts need to remember their backs when sawing wood or working at a bench. The wood should be at the correct level to be sawn without stress. The bench should be high enough for drilling and other operations to be carried out in an upright position. If these activities have to be continued for long periods, then regular rests should be taken, with a little walking around to loosen up the muscles.

If Decorating make sure that the work is being done at a convenient height to cause minimum stress on the back. Unnecessary reaching should be avoided, and never be kept up for long periods. If the ceiling has to be painted, the trestles should be arranged so that the area can be reached with the minimum of stretching and bending. It is better to rearrange the trestles at short intervals than reach out and pull a back muscle. Stop frequently to rest the back, neck and shoulders.

Avoid twisting the body into awkward shapes in order to reach difficult corners.

Gardeners in particular should think BACK before they act. What should be a pleasant and healthy pastime can become a great cause of pain, especially for the elderly. When digging a bed of heavy soil, do not do too much at a time. The soil should be moved by lifting the spade with a straight back and never twist the body to deliver the soil alongside. Take a rest every half hour. Try something else for a while to relax the muscles, returning to the digging later.

Weeding and sowing seeds can be very 'back break-ing'. Instead of bending over, kneel down on a pad or plank, or use a low stool, moving along the bed with-out stretching. Again take regular rests.

Never take off a coat or sweater as the work warms up the body. Chilling the muscles when under stress only increases the risk of damage.

Avoid sudden movements and jumping down from ladders. If a load has to be carried use a wheelbarrow, keeping the handles close to the body when wheeling and never overload the barrow. If a sack of fertiliser has to be carried – and sacks are invariably supplied in quantities which are dangerous to lift singly – try and get help. If not, break down the journey by putting a table or stool halfway. Remember the rules for lifting, carry the sack close to the body and place it on the table for a rest. If it is a long distance, lift it from the table onto the shoulders. Never walk any distance with a heavy sack held in the arms with back bent.

Use long-handled tools for cultivating, and hold them close to the body. When mowing, keep the handles of the lawnmower close to the body so that the back is erect.

How many elderly people have walked around their garden and then seen a weed and quickly bent down to remove it – and ooch! Backache. This is not surprising when we think about our spine. Degeneration has made the spine less flexible and the discs are already compressed. We have provided no exercise to strengthen the supporting muscles, yet we bend suddenly, with a quick jerky movement, probably twisting the body at the same time. Our compressed discs cannot stand the extra strain. We either get a sudden tearing of a ligament or muscle with immediate pain – possibly combined with a spasm of the muscle in self-defence so that we cannot even move – or we think that we are alright and then later in the day perhaps, we sneeze whilst watching television and the disc bulges on to a nerve, and we have weeks of excruciating pain. It is our own fault for not remembering that our spine will take so much stress, and no more. We must learn before it is too late, and to think BACK before we act.

Sportsmen, and women, and those who have enjoyed sports in their youth should also take care of their backs. Osteopaths say that they can always recognise someone who has been a keen rower, as they usually need special treatment in later life. Only recently research has shown that water skiers subject their spines to considerable stress. We all read of golfers, cricketers, tennis players, skiers and other famous sportsmen and women who have had to retire due to back troubles. Some sports put more strain on the back than others, but more care when training, as well as when playing, might have saved them. Fortunately today there are many medical disciplines specialising in back pain available to sportsmen and women.

When we grow older and have to stop our sporting activities it is essential that we continue to exercise our muscles that have been developed in our youth. Otherwise these muscles will lose tone and become rigid, giving less support for the spine. Much of our fine physique will also turn to fat, and if we are not careful we start adding extra fat to the weight that our spines must carry, so that less additional stress is needed to produce backache.

If we start less demanding pastimes in later life, then we must prepare our muscles and body for them. If we are to take up golf for the first time, or even bowls, we should prepare the muscles of the spine for the extra stresses before they occur, or we shall suffer. It is probable that regular daily exercises become more important in later life when this degeneration is making itself felt. It only needs a few minutes exercise night and morning, especially in the morning, to tune up muscles and make the body more flexible, and so avoid stresses on muscles and ligaments.

A word of warning here. If you are a back pain sufferer, do check with your medical adviser to ensure that you are carrying out the correct exercises, as the wrong ones could do more damage than good. There is also a trend these days for 'group exercising', such as 'aerobics' to reduce weight. Make sure that you build up your exercises slowly, doing a little more each day. Do not try and keep up with a class at your first attempt.

Driving is in itself an occupational hazard. We sit in seats which for the most part have not been designed with the spine in mind. There are today a few more advanced car manufacturers who are designing seats with some guidance from back pain specialists, but they are few in number. We are often in one position for hours on end, while suffering the natural stresses of driving which will tend to tighten our muscles. In addition, we may also be suffering some jarring of the spine via the buttocks when the shock-absorbing system is not of the best.

To reduce this stress on the spine by a rather unnatural phenomenon, sit as upright as possible with a cushion or pad in the small of the back (the lumbar region) to give some support. Keep the knees just above the seat with legs out straight to reach the pedals, in a comfortable position. Do not get too close to the pedals with the legs and knees drawn up close to the body. Adjust your seat until the most comfortable position, and rake, is obtained. If driving for long periods, pull off the road every hour or so for a rest. Get out of the car and walk around for a short while to relax the muscles, and relieve your natural tension. Long distance lorry drivers and bus drivers are well known as being major back pain sufferers. We have a chance to avoid this by taking simple precautions.

The foregoing may seem like a series of too many dos and don'ts, but if we think about our back more, the advice given is very simple and only requires a few changes in our habits.

They are all worth remembering, whether a sufferer of backache – when they could reduce further pain – or if one of the lucky ones without back trouble, they will prevent pain in the future.

Chapter 9
Treatments for Back Pain

No advice should be offered to back pain sufferers to deal with their specific complaint in a general manner.
The site and cause of the backache must be carefully diagnosed before any advice or treatment is offered.

Hence, as soon as backache is suffered, the first step must be to visit your general medical practitioner.

As has been stated, pain is personal to the sufferer. He or she can indicate the site of the pain (which may not be the site of the cause) but seldom can he state the extent or nature of that pain, and therefore the medical practitioner cannot always understand the extent of that pain and what it means to the sufferer.

Back pain is often intense, and pain-relieving drugs are frequently used to reduce the suffering, but they can never deal with the cause.

Each medical practitioner will have his own way of identifying and diagnosing the cause of the backache. He has to, because one in every fourteen medical certificates that he signs will be for back trouble.

Many of the more common causes of back trouble are relatively minor, as we have found, and can be treated by rest and pain-relieving drugs. This is therefore, invariably the first treatment given by the general medical practitioner.

In due time if this does not solve the problem, the patient may be sent to a specialist at the local hospital, and X-rays taken so that a more careful diagnosis can be made. Depending on this diagnosis, the treatment may be more rest, traction (the stretching of the body), heat and short wave treatment, massage and exercises or gentle manipulation, all carried out by the hospital physiotherapy department.

It may take a long time for the ligaments, muscles or discs to repair themselves. The sufferer must not be impatient. In many cases it will have taken perhaps many years of misuse of the body to have created the problem, so it cannot be expected to repair itself overnight. Seldom is surgery needed to relieve back pain. Correct diagnosis and treatment will usually work successfully – in time.

In addition to the treatments provided within the Health Service by the medical practitioner, the hospital will have specialist orthopaedic consultants who, with their physiotherapists, will have amassed considerable knowledge and experience for dealing with back problems.

Unorthodox Treatments

In addition, there are other disciplines specialising in problems of the spine. These are Osteopaths and Chiropractors, who use manipulation and often also include at their clinics acupuncture and naturopathy within their treatments.

These specialists outside the Health Service have to be paid for and attended privately. Many back pain sufferers will testify that the only relief or cure they obtained was as a result of treatments by such practitioners. If unorthodox treatment is required, and they can now be recommended by the general medical practitioner, it is wise to ensure that it is given by a qualified registered practitioner. A list of such practitioners can be obtained from their professional association (see page 64). Unfortunately, in many of these unorthodox fields unqualified practitioners are still permitted to practice.

There are also medically-qualified specialists in private practice, such as orthopaedic surgeons, rheumatologists, doctors and physiotherapists who have also recieved training in osteopathy and chiropractic. Some other doctors also practice manipulative treatment similar to osteopaths and chiropractors, and offer a private service.

The Use of 'Orthopaedic'

It is perhaps appropriate here to give a word of warning. Since backache has become a 'popular' malady in recent years, a few manufacturers of bedding and seating have 'borrowed' the term 'orthopaedic' to provide special bedding and seating for back pain sufferers, usually at high cost, which some claim will solve all back troubles.

As has been shown, there are many causes of backache, all requiring different treatments. No one bed or chair can solve all backache problems, nor be suitable for all sufferers, although some may give a degree of relief for some of the milder forms of backache.

When buying a new bed, the recommendation is to shop around carefully and test the mattress before buying. Often a board placed between mattress and base will give the necessary firmness as a temporary measure and be more effective than an 'orthopaedic' bed. The bedding industry is now attempting to grade mattresses from soft (No 1) to firm (No 6), so that the grade of firmness can be selected to suit the buyer best. Some back pain sufferers find a soft bed preferable to a firm grade. What must be avoided is an old mattress which sags, as this provides no support whatever to the spine.

Similarly with chairs, support in the lumbar region may be required, and is always recommended rather than a shape which encourages slouching. Often however, a pad or cushion will suffice rather than an 'orthopaedic' chair. It is better to choose a comfortable chair that encourages sitting upright, than a special chair in which it is impossible to relax. Many back pain specialists recommend the use of rocking chairs.

Exercises

Exercises can be used to give relief from many forms of backache by strengthening the muscles, creating greater flexibility, providing traction and generally creating better posture and movement. There are many books of such exercises, and even a tape setting these exercises to music which is obtainable from the National Back Pain Association (see page 64) It must be repeated, however, that you should always consult your medical practitioner, osteopath or chiropractor to ensure that the exercises are suitable for you. The wrong type of exercise could do damage and certainly give no relief. For this reason no specific exercises are recommended here.

Chapter 10
Conclusion and Prevention
Check List

In this little book I have tried to give some helpful advice so that sufferers from backache will understand the nature of their problem, and will have derived some hope in that most cases backache, whilst often very painful, is not likely to be permanent, is never terminal and that much can be done to relieve the suffering.

For those who have had an occasional twinge, or may not have suffered at all, I have given some warnings. If they think BACK before they act they can live happily without suffering backache at all. Prevention is possible and is well worthwhile.

The point is made again that with so many different types of back trouble, from different causes and with different effects – each requires different treatment. Accurate diagnosis is essential before any effective treatment can be given. Therefore beware of simple answers and pieces of equipment which are claimed to provide general relief or cure.

Ultimately it relies on sensible use of the body, enjoying sensible activities, maintaining good posture and movement and keeping the correct weight.

Finally, many backache sufferers, having read this little book will be able to understand where they went wrong and so developed spinal trouble. They will wish that they had only known more about their spine and how to avoid misusing it. It is now up to them to see that others are informed of the dangers and how to avoid them, whilst they themselves learn to live with their backache, taking care not to exacerbate the position.

Here, therefore, are a few useful reminders:

1 S.U.S. Stand up straight, sit up straight.
2 Lift with your legs and arms, not your back.
3 Never lift more than you can manage. Get help.
4 Check that your home, and your work place, is a safe environment.
5 Reduce stress to the minimum.
6 Watch your weight, especially as you age.
7 Carry out regular exercise.
8 Bend over as little as possible.
9 Think BACK, all the time.

Chapter 11
Where to Get Help

First see your general medical practitioner.

If you need additional help, you may care to contact the following organisations. Always enclose a stamped addressed envelope for their reply:

NATIONAL BACK PAIN ASSOCIATION, 31–33 Park Road, Teddington, Middlesex, TW11 OAB.

A registered medical charity devoted to raising funds for back pain research and educating the public on how to avoid back pain. They cannot deal with individual cases, but will send literature about back pain. They have a quarterly magazine and local branches where back pain problems are discussed.

GENERAL COUNCIL & REGISTER OF OSTEOPATHS, 21 Suffolk Street, London W1Y 4HG

BRITISH CHIROPRACTORS ASSOCIATION, Premier House, 10 Greycoat Place, London SW1P 1SB

ACUPUNCTURE REGISTER & DIRECTORY OF PRACTITIONERS 34 Alderney Street, Pimlico, London SW1V 4EU

BRITISH ASSOCIATION OF MANIPULATIVE MEDICINE
30a Wimpole Street, London W1M 7AE

BRITISH ORTHOPAEDIC ASSOCIATION c/o Royal College
of Surgeons, Lincoln's Inn Fields, London WC2

BRITISH HOMEOPATHIC ASSOCIATION 27a Devonshire
Street, London W1N 1RJ

ORGANISATION OF CHARTERED PHYSIOTHERAPISTS IN
PRIVATE PRACTICE c/o 14 Bedford Row, London WC1R
4ED

LONDON COLLEGE OF OSTEOPATHIC MEDICINE
8–10 Boston Place, London W1

CHIROPRACTIC ADVANCEMENT ASSOCIATION 56 Barnes
Crescent, Wimborne, Dorset BH21 1AZ

Acknowledgments

Back Pain Association: Lifting Posters, 'Think Back'

The Back, Relief From Pain by Dr Alan Stoddard

Two Four Letter Words: Back Pain by Dr S.K. Manstead

Avoiding Back Trouble from Consumers Association

My thanks go to these recognised specialists in back pain:
Dr S.T. Pheasant PhD, of the Department of Anatomy at The Royal Free Hospital and
Mr Chris Hayne FCSP, of the Physiotherapy Department of The Derbyshire Royal Infirmary, for their careful checking of the medical facts contained in this brief summary on backpain, its causes and how to avoid it.

Notes

Keep a record of any back pain attacks, and the treatment given, for possible repetition later. As will have been seen, back pain is likely to repeat itself if considerable care is not taken.